HEALTHY DIET

FOR A

HEALTHY LIFE

Everything You Need to Know About Eating for a
Healthy Life.

RITA LUCKY

Conditions of Use

The Publisher has attempted to be as accurate and complete as possible in the creation of this report, notwithstanding the fact that, due to the rapidly changing nature of the Internet, she does not warrant or represent at any time that the contents contained within are accurate.

While every effort has been made to verify the information in this publication, the Publisher accepts no responsibility for errors, omissions, or contrary interpretations of the subject matter contained herein. Any perceived slights against specific individuals, groups, or organizations are unintentional.

There are no income guarantees in practical advice books, as there are in anything else in life. Readers are advised to base their responses on their own personal experiences.

This book is not a source of legal, business, accounting, or financial advice. All readers are advised to seek the advice of competent professionals in the fields of law, business, accounting, and finance.

This book is recommended for printing for ease of reading.

Contents Table

Chapter 1

The Fundamentals

Chapter 2

The Way You Think About Food

Chapter 3

Honey And Whole Grains

Chapter 4

Nuts And Lean Meat

Chapter 5

The Benefits

Final Thoughts

Foreword

Simply put, the body has two very different and complex systems for producing energy. Because energy is essential to human activity and survival, the two-energy style relies on each other for support. This book explains which foods provide the most energy.

It happens all the time: we decide to start a health and fitness program with zeal and, most likely, fanfare; however, in the first few weeks, everything fails as a result of going into the plan.

Why don't we stick to the diet plans, morning jogging plans, and physical exercise plans that we devise?

And what can we do to ensure that we stick to our plans, both for our own sake and for the sake of those who rely on us?

Are you eating to satisfy your hunger or to please your taste buds? Or are you eating to gain more control over your life? In this eBook, we will look at how you can improve your life simply by eating correctly.

Healthy Diet for a healthy life

DEDICATION

This book is dedicated to God Almighty for the knowledge given to me to compile this book, to my late dad Mr. Rapheal who thought me a whole lot on eating to live up to 100years and plus.

Chapter 1

Energy is required for a variety of functions such as growth maintenance, daily activities, exercise, and a variety of other movements or functions that are frequently overlooked. These are shared by both energy systems.

In today's world, few health and fitness plans are successful. What is the cause of their alarming failure rate?

The world today is far less healthy than it was two decades ago. Much of this is due to people's changing eating habits.

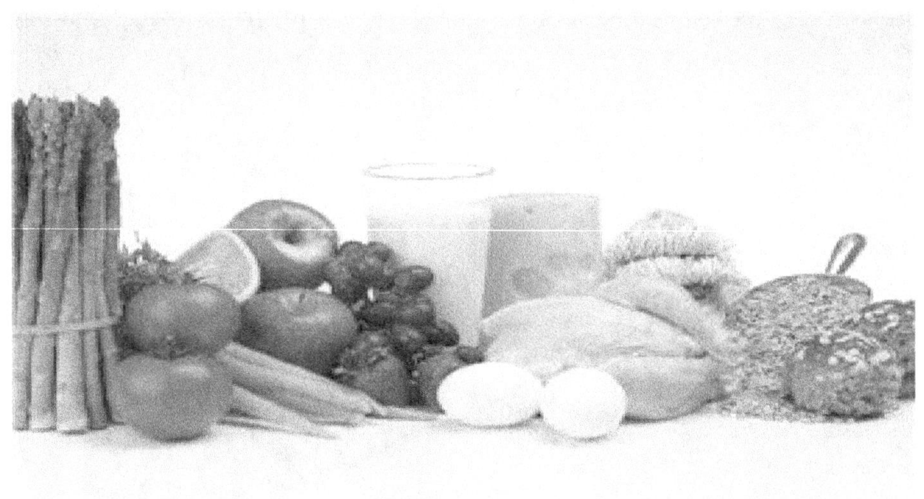

The aerobic system is the primary and first to be used energy system. This system requires a lot from the body in order for the muscles to function properly.

This demand typically increases the rate and depth of breathing as well as blood supply, owing to the corresponding increase in heart rate.

When the body requires more energy and this cannot be met due to the increased need for more oxygen, the body system switches to anaerobic energy. This system can generate energy without the use of oxygen.

All of this energy is generated by the appropriate or correct consumption of foods. The foods consumed determine the types of energy levels that each person is capable of producing.

Muscle fatigue typically occurs when all energy sources are depleted, which can be attributed to a number of factors, the most compelling of which is the type of foods consumed.

There are several food categories that produce various beneficial elements for the human body system, with the ones that create or enhance energy generating sources being of particular interest is definitely helpful to know. As a result, this knowledge should assist the individual in selecting the appropriate types of foods.

The aerobic system works by breaking down the carbohydrates, fatty acids, and amino acids in the foods we eat, whereas the anaerobic system releases energy from the foods we store in our bodies, usually during periods of intense activity.

If we hear about diets or gym plans failing all around us, it's usually not their fault. It is usually the fault of the people who made a big deal out of going through these plans, telling all their friends and co-workers about it and then failed to adhere to those programs.

Individuals who abandon the exercise or diet program in the middle do not see the benefits, and everyone blames the plan.

What the world requires today is motivation, not a new health or fitness program or diet. It takes the right kind of mindset to see through whatever plan they have chosen to the end.

If they can accomplish this, most health issues associated with lifestyle will become obsolete. And we don't have to travel to the ends of the earth to find this motivation. The motivation is right here, within us; we just need to find it and use it.

A generation ago, people would not have dreamed of eating whatever junk food they could get their hands on. Nowadays, we do it so casually. "I'm hungry," in most cases, means "I want a burger or a hot dog, probably with chips and cola on the side." And "I'm on a diet" means "I'm on a chemically laced pill that will satisfy my hunger while depriving my body of vitamins."

It's no surprise that we have so many health problems today.

Our health is a reflection of the foods we eat. The sorry state in which we find ourselves is not an individual issue; it is a global one. The entire world is eating incorrectly. Six out of every ten people in the United States is overweight, and by 2025, eight out of every ten people will be overweight.

Are we really considering this? We aren't. Even if you're reading this eBook, you're probably snacking on some chips. Do you realize that the money you spent on that package, which is filling your stomach with some of the most toxic chemicals known to humanity, could have fed an undernourished child in Ruanda?

But it's not just about being generous. It's also about us. Yes, we must be self-centered. With such dismal health statistics, aren't we on the verge of disaster? We're definitely not eating properly. We must be prepared for whatever excess baggage that brings, such as obesity and other ill health consequences - we have to be prepared for it.

So, the next time you see a program that has failed or is receiving a lot of criticism, remember that it isn't because the program is on shaky ground. In most cases, it is because people began with good intentions but then did not adhere to the program as strictly as they should have.

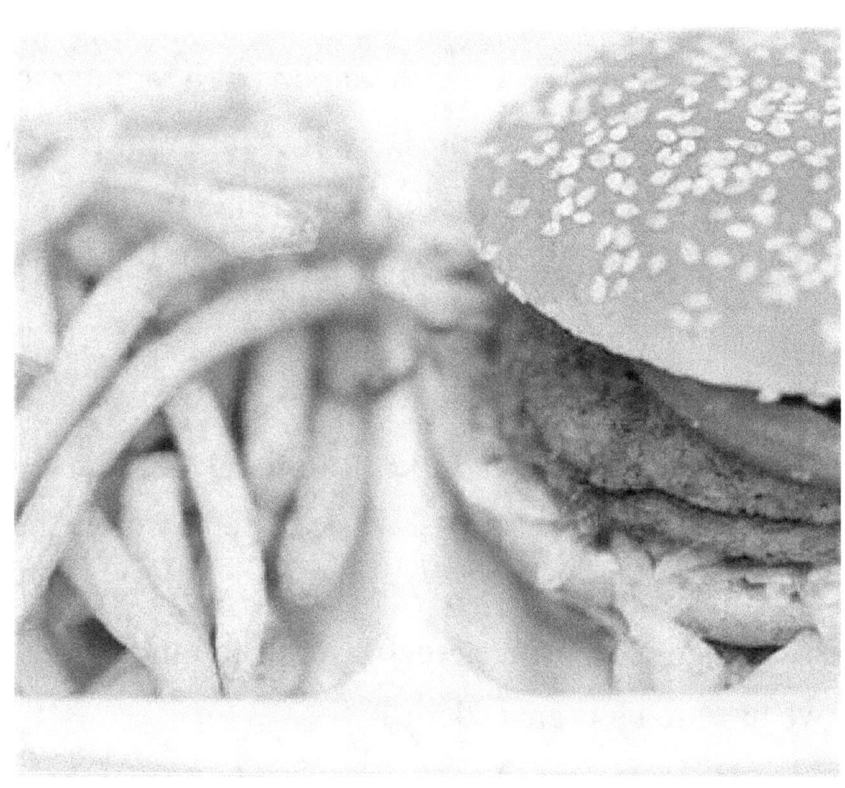

Chapter 2

The most important thing you need to keep your health and fitness program going – even more important than an instructor or a doctor – is your own motivation.

You must be determined to investigate the situation. So, you're a little overweight and want to lose a few pounds. No gym instructor in the world will be able to help you if you do not take the necessary steps to maintain a healthy diet and adhere to a regular exercise regimen.

Even if you're sick and considering treatment, no doctor will be able to help you if you're not committed to following the treatment plan, whether it's taking the medication at the right time or avoiding certain foods.

So far, our eating habits have been disastrous. Things will not improve unless we take stock of the situation and take control of the situation.

The most important factor is awareness. We must learn which foods are good for us and which are not. We must return to training to determine which nutrients your body requires and in what quantities.

Then we must devise a dietary regimen for ourselves and our loved ones in order to eat healthier. We must eliminate all harmful foods - sugars, fats, and carbohydrates, which we do not desire - and replace them with foods that may benefit our health.

I understand if this sounds too preachy. But that is the only respite we have. We'll never be able to improve if we keep eating Oreos.

But there is still hope. There are a lot of foods out there that are just as tasty as those horrible junk foods, but we don't know about them yet.

These are the foods that we aren't aware of because we don't like them or don't know how to prepare them, but a healthy cookbook may assist you in comprehending various intriguing approaches to healthy cooking.

Even if you stick to the same diet, you can create some really delicious healthy dishes. Yes, everything is possible. You can significantly alter your eating habits while also paying attention to your palate.

The truth is that the weight loss industry has played a significant role in the decline of the developed human race. They must continue to sell Atkins, Jenny Craig, Zones, and Medi fasts as a result, the media never tells you how we can actually take matters into our own hands.

They show us glitzy before-and-after pictures of a person with a foot-long sub and then the same guy with six pack abs and tell us that the diet allowed them to achieve that.

However, if we put our heads together, we could easily do that as well, without having to spend thousands of dollars on those diets. And what should we do?

2 Broad Points: -

    i)   Control what we eat.

    ii)   Engage in some physical activity.

Is that too much to ask of you? Don't we owe it to our bodies, which have served us so well over the years? Isn't that something we owe to ourselves and our loved ones?

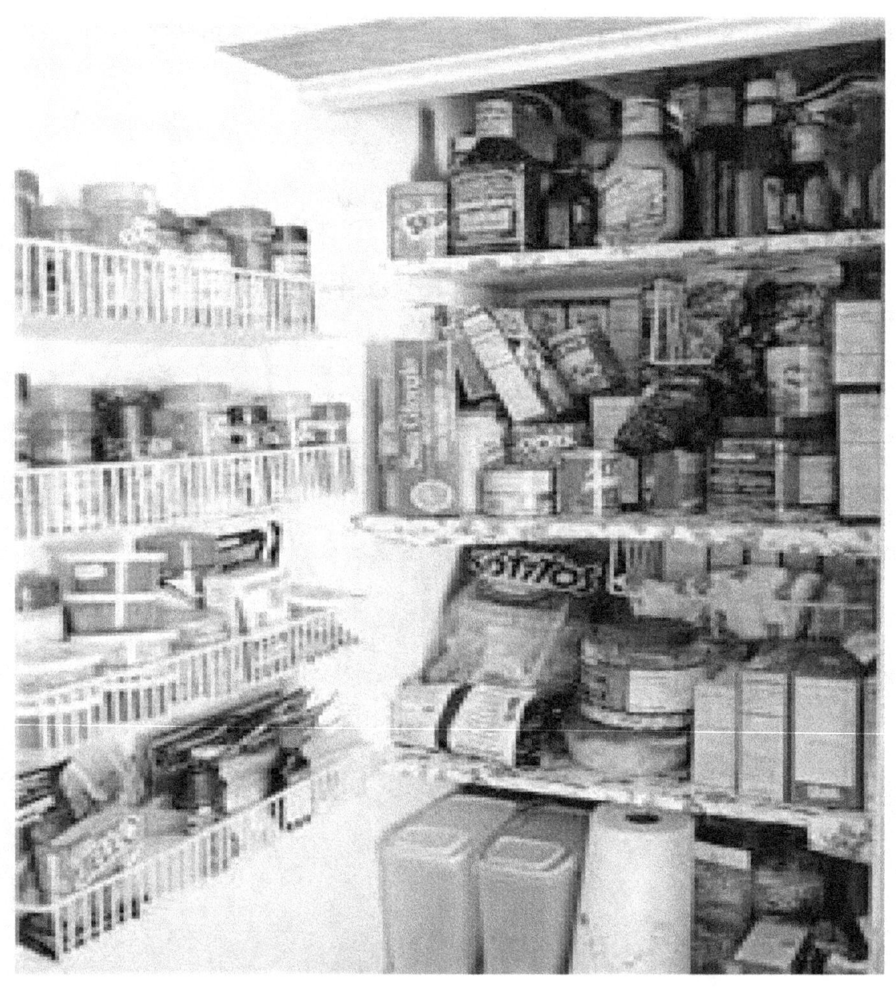

Chapter 3

Honey has been shown to be a sustaining power behind the energy circle over time. It benefits the human body in a variety of ways, but it is most notable for its ability to produce energy. Honey is nature's most natural source of energy. It also serves as an effective immune system booster, as well as a natural remedy for a variety of ailments.

Energy is critical to the natural flow of any human being's daily life cycle. As a result, finding energy sources that are both consistent and healthy is critical to staying fit and happy.

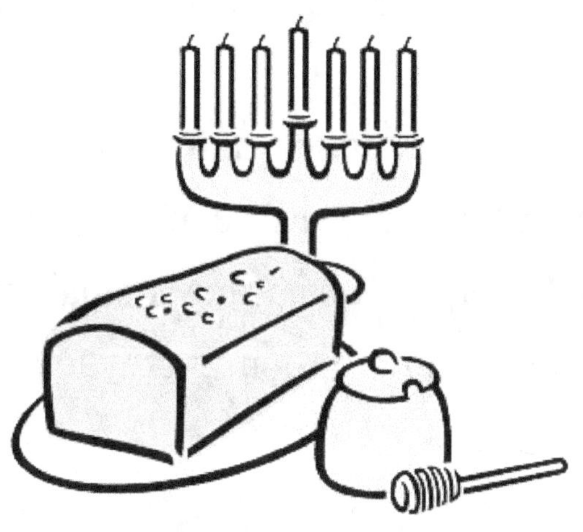

A Perfect Match

Honey's natural benefits are widely recognized and accepted. Aside from its delicious flavor, honey is a natural source of carbohydrate, which is an energy source for improving performance, endurance, and reducing muscle fatigue.

This is especially beneficial to athletes. The sugar content of honey aids in the prevention of fatigue during exercise sessions and training sessions for sports enthusiasts. These sugars are divided into glucose and fructose, which serve different but complementary functions.

The glucose in honey is generally absorbed faster and provides an immediate energy boost, whereas the fructose works at a slower rate and provides a more sustainable and prolonged energy dispersant. When it comes to blood sugar levels in the body, honey has been shown to help keep them relatively constant.

Consuming honey is not a difficult exercise because it is a pleasant food product that is natural in its form. People of all ages are generally eager to consume honey in any of its associated forms. It's even popular among kids.

Consuming a small amount of honey daily provides energy to children, allowing them to cope with the physical demands of daily school activities as well as sports commitments. Consuming a small amount of honey on a daily basis can help adults maintain their energy levels during a long day at work.

Making sandwiches with honey and other fillings is one way to make a tasty snack. A freshly toasted slice of bread with honey on top is also a tasty breakfast option. Using honey instead of sugar in drinks is strongly encouraged.

Most people today want a quick fix for their energy needs, which usually comes in the form of unhealthy sports drinks, coffee, and refined carbohydrates such as sugar and white bread.

Though these produce the desired increased energy levels, it should be noted that this energy is relatively fleeting, and the tiredness that follows is usually more acutely felt. Consuming some form of whole grains is thus not only a better option, but also much healthier.

Whole grains provide energy in a more complex form that degrades over a longer period of time. This then serves as the foundation for maintaining energy levels for longer periods of time.

Because of their more complex composition, whole grains contain a variety of beneficial elements such as minerals, vitamins, phytonutrients, and fiber.

Including whole grain ingredients in any dish almost always completes or enhances the flavor. Whole grains include wheat, oat, barley, maize, brown rice, faro, spelt, emmer, einkorn, rye, millet, buckwheat, and many others.

These can then be processed into whole wheat flour, whole wheat bread, whole wheat pasta, rolled oats or oat groats, triticale flour, popcorn, and teff flour.

Consuming whole grains on a regular basis can help reduce the risk of heart disease, lower cholesterol levels, protect against many types of cancer, and aid in weight management. Whole grains should not be confused with their less refined "cousin." Though refined grains have some advantages, whole grain alternatives are always preferable.

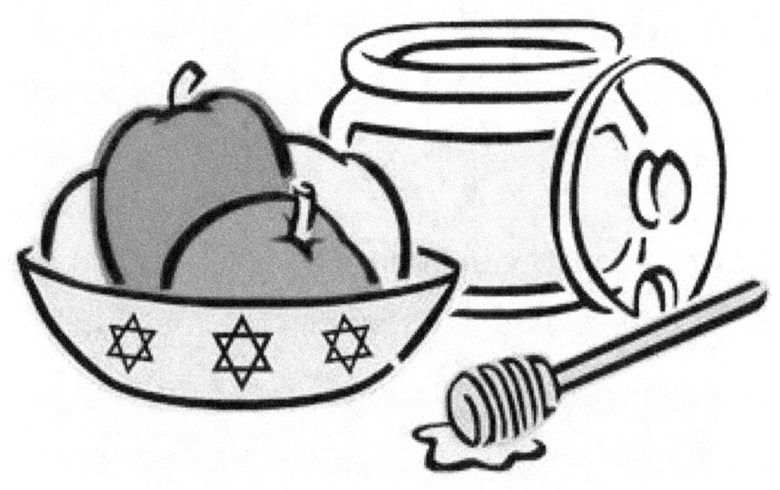

Chapter 4

Nuts are a valuable source of nutrients for both humans and animals. It is high in a variety of essential nutrients and can be consumed raw, cooked, or as an addition to pre-existing dishes. Though nuts are defined as a hard-shelled fruit, there are many other foods that are included in the nut family.

Different types of meat contribute to a wide range of flavors; however, the healthiest type contains as much lean meat as possible. It is undeniable that meats with a high fat content are delicious, but for health reasons, taking the time to understand the benefits of eating lean meats is extremely prudent.

Proteins And Oils That Are Nutritious

It is now widely accepted that nuts can significantly reduce or prevent the occurrence of many ailments. For example, nuts have been shown to reduce the likelihood of coronary heart disease manifesting, even in people who come from a long line of affected family members.

Consuming nuts such as almonds and walnuts has been shown to lower serum cholesterol levels in the body. Nuts are also highly recommended for people who have insulin resistance issues, such as diabetics.

Another healthier option is to satisfy cravings with nuts rather than junk food. Another advantage of choosing nuts as a healthier alternative is that they contain essential fatty acids. Because nuts are nutritious and can be eaten raw, they are an excellent snack to keep on hand.

Because of their slow burn characteristics, which help to keep blood sugar levels consistently healthy, almonds are frequently used to normalize blood lipids. The almond is a popular addition to the stale diet of most Mediterranean people because it is high in a variety of nutrients.

The Brazil nut is another nutritious nut that has its own set of advantages when consumed in moderation. The Brazil nut is high in omega 3 fatty acids and a good source of calcium.

Another popular nut that is frequently consumed as a salted snack is the cashew nut. However, without the addition of salt, it would be a much healthier food product, as it is already a flavorful nut on its own. These nuts are processed into oils in some parts of the world.

The selection process should be done with limited knowledge because relying solely on what the naked eye perceives is insufficient. Round, chuck, sirloin, and tenderloin are examples of lean beef cuts, while tenderloin, loin chops, and leg are examples of lean pork or lamb cuts. The breast area without the skin is the leanest part of the poultry.

Though there are many reasons why people avoid eating meat on a daily basis, there is no evidence that this is a good or bad choice that should be followed by everyone.

The important point to note here is the selection of the types of meats that would make consumption healthy, which would generally mean meats with lower fat content. Though white meat is not without fat, it is significantly lower in fat content than red meats.

Consuming lean meats has a wide range of nutritional benefits. Lean meats have a higher and purer protein content, which is an important factor in the fundamental structural and functional progress of every cell sustenance and formation.

Lean meats are also high in essential amino acids, especially sulfur amino acids. When compared to the digestive rates, meat proteins work faster than those found in beans and whole wheat.

Iron is also abundant in lean meat. Because iron deficiency is progressive, it is frequently not detected until anemia has developed.

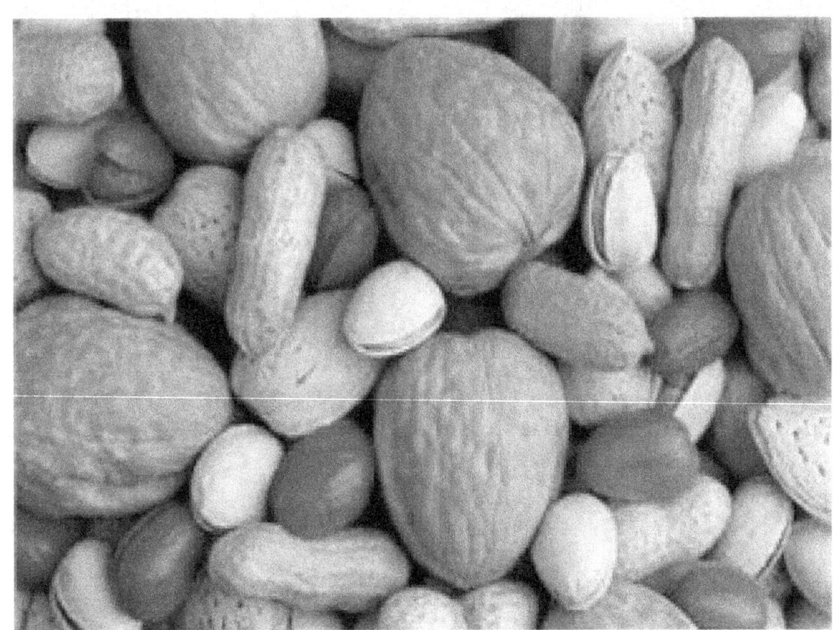

Chapter 5

The Benefits

Here is all the motivation you need to keep eating healthy.

Let's get right into the meat of the matter.

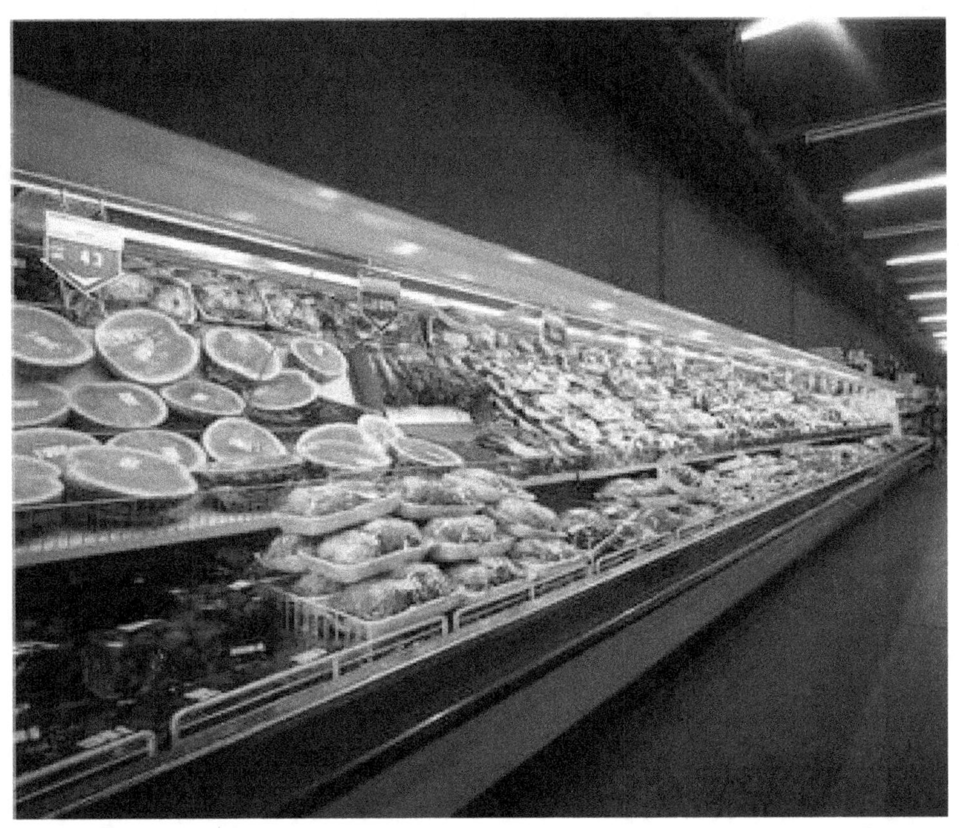

Advantages

You Improve Your Health

We could read a whole library of books about the health benefits of eating properly and still not cover what benefits truly exist. The most significant benefit is that you gain control over your weight.

By eating correctly, you also ensure that your metabolic functions, particularly your immune and gastrointestinal systems, continue to function properly. You are also protected from a variety of chronic diseases, including cardiovascular diseases such as coronary artery disease and high blood pressure, as well as diabetes.

More inexpensive

Eating healthily saves you money. Your supermarket bills drop dramatically, and you avoid furthering your charge card debt if you already have one. Furthermore, you save a significant amount of money on all of the healthcare costs that would be incurred if an issue arose as a result of your food binging habits.

Less toxins in your body

Many foods today are toxic due to the presence of synthetic chemicals. When you try to eat correctly, you are much less likely to get these toxins into your body because one of the basic dogmas of eating correctly is that you should avoid eating anything man-made.

Furthermore, if you eat less, you will be able to cut back on vices such as smoking and alcoholism. A glass of beer is almost always associated with a night out with the guys. If you eat less, you won't crave beer as much. Similarly, you will not want to have that one (or more) mandatory smoke after each meal.

Increased physical activity

When you eat better, you'll notice that you can do your job much better. You can exercise more, travel more, play more, and work more, making your life more productive.

That sure beat being a slob and lounging on the couch all day, doesn't it? You can also be more involved with your friends and loved ones, which will undoubtedly enrich your life.

Affluent Social Life

Forget about fat fetishism; people who are overweight do not appear attractive. Weight on the wrong parts of the body is frowned upon in society. If you're looking for a partner, your flab could be an issue.
Not only that, but people who can't control their eating habits and thus their weight are viewed negatively by society as people who can't control

their basic urges.

This type of psychology does exist, but very few people will discuss it. When you eat properly, you'll notice that these problems go away.

Final Thoughts

There are numerous popular diets on the market today, but the majority of them are unhealthy and, in some cases, dangerous. This will teach you how to eat a healthy, balanced diet for life and avoid unhealthy diets.

Determine how many calories your body requires each day to function.

This number can vary greatly depending on your metabolism and level of physical activity. If you're the type of person who gains ten pounds just by smelling a slice of pizza, your daily caloric intake should be around 2000 calories for men and 1500 calories for women.

Your body mass index also plays a role: more calories are appropriate for naturally larger individuals, and fewer calories are appropriate for naturally smaller individuals. If you can eat without gaining weight or are physically active, you may want to increase your daily caloric intake by 1000-2000 calories, slightly less for women.

Don't be afraid of fatty foods.

For your body to function properly, you must consume fat from foods. However, it is critical to select the right kinds of fats: Most animal fats and a few vegetable oils are high in the type of fat that raises LDL cholesterol; the bad cholesterol.

Unlike popular belief, eating cholesterol does not increase the amount of cholesterol in your body. If you give your body the right tools, it will flush out excess cholesterol. These are monounsaturated fatty acids, which you should try to consume on a regular basis. Olive oil, nuts, fish oil, and various seed oils are high in monounsaturated fatty acids.

Consume plenty of the right carbs.

You must consume carbohydrates because they are your body's primary source of energy. The trick is to choose the right carbs. Simple carbohydrates, such as sugar and refined flour, are quickly absorbed by the gastrointestinal system.

This causes a type of carb overload, and your body responds by releasing massive amounts of insulin to combat the overload. Excess insulin not only harms your heart, but it also promotes weight gain. Consume plenty of carbohydrates, but choose carbohydrates that are slowly digested by the body, such as whole grain flour, vegetables, oats, and unprocessed grains.

Eat larger meals first thing in the morning.

Your metabolism slows down toward the end of the evening and your digestion becomes less efficient. This means that more of the energy stored in food will be stored as fat, and your body will not absorb as many nutrients from the meal. Breakfast should be medium-sized, lunch should be large, and dinner should be small. Better yet, try eating 4-6 small meals throughout the day.

Make a cheat meal for yourself.

Cheating does not imply bingeing on all the wrong foods once a week; rather, it means enjoying a food you truly enjoy once a week. On Sundays, have a couple slices of pizza, and on Saturdays, have a huge slice of double chocolate cake. This cheat meal will help you stick to your diet change and is beneficial to your body in a few ways. Cheat meals include special occasions such as family birthdays.

Make it a habit to eat slowly.

It will satisfy you with fewer calories and will prevent overeating and obesity, as well as all of their consequences.

Drink plenty of water.

It makes you feel more awake and energized, improves your skin, and makes you feel fuller, so you eat less! Cutting back on soda and replacing it with water will benefit you greatly.

www.ingramcontent.com/pod-product-compliance
Lightning Source LLC
Chambersburg PA
CBHW081405160726
48000CB00010B/3488